Intermittent Fasting: Beginner's Guide to Losing Weight, Increasing Longevity, and Improving your Immune System

Copyright 2018 - All rights reserved.

This document is geared towards providing exact and reliable information in regards to the topic and issue covered. The publication is sold with the idea that the publisher is not required to render an accounting, officially permitted, or otherwise, qualified services. If advice is necessary, legal or professional, a practiced individual in the profession should be ordered.

- From a Declaration of Principles which was accepted and approved equally by a Committee of the American Bar Association and a Committee of Publishers and Associations.

Table of Contents

Introduction

I would like to take this opportunity to thank you for purchasing this book: "Intermittent Fasting: Beginner's Guide to Losing Weight, Increasing Longevity, and improving your Immune System."

In case you have already heard of intermittent fasting, but don't know how it works, this is the perfect book for you. During the course of this book, you will learn how Intermittent Fasting works, how beneficial it is and to make it simple for you; I have suggested dietary chart plans. Many consider the idea of intermittent fasting as a difficult task or an unsafe method, which could cause complications to their health. Though there are side effects associated with this method, it gets serious only when the person using this type of fast is not careful about choosing his diet protocol. Therefore, it is crucial to understand Intermittent Fasting before you practice it.

Intermittent fasting is simple when compared to other fasting methods. You need to fast for the prescribed period of time, and then consume the calories required for your body during the eating window. This eating window can be for six to eight hours on an average in a day. Does it sound unhealthy or uncomfortable to you? Well, it isn't. This fasting method is a useful tool to improve your dietary compliance. Many people who had already practiced intermittent fasting enjoy the method more than the traditional eating patterns people use in this day and age. This is because it allows you to have larger meals during the eating window.

Have you been struggling to lose weight for a long time? Then this book has the perfect solution for you. Intermittent fasting can help you lose weight by getting rid of that extra fat and flab on your body. You need to ensure you fit this fasting method into your regular routine in the right way. Choose a well-balanced approach that will work best for your body type, lifestyle and health goals.

It is crucial to know how to make intermittent fasting work best for your body. You should be able to get your work style, daily routine and eating habits in place. It can be pretty tricky to follow the fasting method due to the following criteria:

- Your exercise routine
- Your meal time
- Your work routine, etc

While intermittent fasting, you need to make exercise a priority and, at the same time, eat better.

In this book, we will discuss what intermittent fasting is, its role to help lose weight and the various other benefits it provides. It is essential to enjoy the positive aspects of this diet, as it is good for your mind and body. The chapters in this book will help you understand more about intermittent fasting, the various fasting methods and the ways to get started. The chapters will also talk about how to boost your immune system and increase longevity.

I hope this book serves as an informative and interesting!

Happy Reading!

Chapter One: Brief About Intermittent Fasting

Do you want to lose weight?

- Ensure you start your day with a healthy breakfast, as it provides the required energy to kick start your day. Eat breakfast like a king, lunch like a prince and dinner like a pauper.

- Ensure you have six small meals spread throughout the day. This will give your body the required energy and strength to function properly for the entire day.

There is research and various studies that show that people who eat earlier in the day lose more weight when compared to the ones who eat late breakfast or skip a meal. The moral of the story – Eat breakfast to lose weight and have a healthy body!

Done? Is that all? No, not really. There is much more to the story. It is important to concentrate on your mental and physical health by devising a proper diet plan. The diet chart should not just concentrate on losing your body fat or gaining muscle mass; it should work toward optimal performance.

Many people have a lot of questions about weight loss, especially after hearing about intermittent fasting from their friends or family members. They will want answers to all their queries, such as:

- Is it necessary to fast for 24 hours on an occasional basis?
- What is the 16/8 intermittent fasting protocol all about?

- Will I be able to fast with my odd working hours?
- Does this fasting method really work?
- Will it work differently on men and women?
- Should I keep a strict check on my calories?

The first and foremost thing you need to understand about intermittent fasting is that it is not a diet but a dieting pattern. This means the fasting method allows you to make a conscious decision to skip specific meals on purpose – be it breakfast, lunch or dinner. It completely depends on the protocol you choose.

When you fast and then eat during a particular period, you tend to consume calories during a specific time interval of the day and not to eat for the remaining period of the day. This automatically reduces your calorie consumption, as your eating period is less when compared to your fasting period. There are various ways to take advantage of the intermittent fasting method.

Intermittent Fasting

Intermittent fasting will include different varieties of dieting methods that focus on shuffling between periods of not eating and eating. When you look at the usual fasting methods, you will mostly fast for the whole day or eat only one meal a day. But this is not the case with intermittent fasting. You will actually be eating every day of the week. The only thing you should remember is not what you eat, but when you eat.

Your eating time is scheduled in a strict pattern and severely restricted. The calorie intake is also reduced to a much lower level when compared to your normal eating routine. There are many different ways to approach intermittent fasting.

For instance, a few people go by the traditional approach of not eating in the morning and have a small meal in the evening. But there are a few others who will have a large meal in the morning and starve for the rest of the day. Some people may have a regular diet one day and then go on a daylong fast the next day. There might also be people who will have a week of normal eating with one day of intermittent fasting.

The fasting pattern completely depends on the person who is going to follow the diet. There are so many varieties when it comes to intermittent fasting. This fasting method has one of the most useful and interesting dieting patterns. But people who generally follow the intermittent fasting approach don't eat for sixteen hours in a day.

Basic approach

Though there are many types of intermittent fasting methods, it is better to understand the basic method to give you an idea of how it works. The most commonly used intermittent fasting method is the 16/8 approach. Using this method, a person can have an eating window of eight hours during which they can choose to have one meal or have more meals spread across in that time limit.

You don't need to limit the choice of food you eat, as the calories will, by default, be less than normal. But, it is always advisable to keep a check on the food you choose. For instance, eating complete junk or oily food or red meat or dairy products during the eating window will not do you any good.

Once you finish this eight-hour eating period, you will have to fast for sixteen hours. This might sound challenging but is actually not that hard. You need to make sure you approach the format reasonably.

For instance, out of the sixteen hours fasting period, you can use the eight-hour sleeping time as a part of your intermittent fasting chart. Technically speaking, you will have to eat four hours before you sleep and then eat four hours after you wake up. Sleep time will be eight hours. So, 4 hours (before sleep) + 4 hours (after sleep) + 8 hours (during sleep) will complete your sixteen hours fasting window.

One more important thing you need to remember when intermittent fasting is that you are allowed to have plenty of liquids during your fasting window. Your body needs to be hydrated during this period. All you need to do is ensure your drinks don't have any calories. You can drink loads of water, fresh cold-pressed juice (without sugar or sweetener), herbal tea (no refined sugar or sweetener), green smoothies (no dairy products), black coffee, etc. It is better to stay away from flavored water or diet sodas during your fasting period.

Though diet sodas don't have any calories, they do carry chemicals that might disturb your fasting process. Always stick to water, herbal tea and black coffee during the fasting window. If you are feeling too hungry or tired, you can have smoothies or juices.

Is fasting new to humans?

Fasting is not new to the human race, as humans have had to fast for numerous reasons since the beginning of their evolution. The ancient cavemen used to fast when they had no food or when food supplies were low. They used to be careful while managing their food and also took in low-calorie foods for the survival of their tribes. Scientifically speaking, the human body is definitely capable of handling fasting methods.

Another interesting fact is that our own body will force us to fast if we are sick due to mild illness or severe disease. This is the reason why we don't feel like eating when we are down with a fever or any form of ailment. The reason for this is quite natural as the body is actually trying to starve out the disease by limiting its calorie intake. It is true that fasting can cause the body to do unusual things, such as increase the immune system, burn the stored fat for energy, etc.

Cultural significance

When people began to develop religious beliefs, fasting was no more just a survival technique. It became a religious ritual. Every major religion in the world has specific fasting methods. For instance, in Catholicism, fasting is observed during the season of Lent. They automatically restrict their meat intake, which leads to less calorie intake in the body.

When it comes to Buddhism, fasting is done to release the body from the need to consume regular food. It also cleanses the mind along with the body. The idea behind this approach is to increase a person's spiritual strength and control the negative urges of the body.

All this information narrows down to the fact that fasting is not dangerous to the body. It is not something new or strange for humans. It is completely acceptable by the human body. Intermittent fasting can have numerous benefits if it is handled properly.

People who have tried intermittent fasting

There have been many athletes and celebrities who have followed the intermittent fasting approach to attain a good physique or get back to shape quickly. This fasting method has grown in popularity and is now used by many people. Let us look at few of the celebrities who have practiced intermittent fasting to get to shape:

Hugh Jackman

The Wolverine compulsively uses intermittent fasting to get into shape and lose that extra weight for his character in the X-Men movie series.

Beyoncé

The popular American singer never fails to use intermittent fasting to get a better body whenever she has to go on a musical tour.

Ben Affleck

The famous American actor claims to have used intermittent fasting to get a good physique whenever he plays action roles, such as in The Daredevil, etc. He says he has seen good results in losing fat using this fasting method especially after he had gained weight for his other acting performances.

Apart from staying in shape, there are many different reasons for using this approach.

A study conducted by New Jersey's University of Medicine and Dentistry revealed that this fasting method helps to:

- Improve immune system
- Manage inflammation
- Reduce the obesity level
- Curb the growth of cancerous tumors

The most surprising factor was – this fasting method could protect the body from many severe types of DNA damage that were caused by environmental toxins.

How does intermittent fasting work?

This super fasting method works by putting your body into a fat-burning phase. This is referred as the ketogenic state. This state basically occurs when your body is low in carbohydrates and is not in a position to convert them into energy using the body's insulin. So, how do you get your energy when you fast?

Since the body has low carbohydrates and cannot convert them to energy, it will turn to the stored fats for energy. This means your body will look for the stored body fat and break it down for energy. This will result in burning all the fat content and help to get you a leaner and healthier body.

Ketogenic diets usually focus on protein-heavy foods and restrict you from consuming sugar and carbohydrates. There are many types of ketogenic diet, and they all come with limitations. But this is not the case with intermittent fasting, as this fasting method doesn't have any restrictions when it comes to what to eat. The reason behind this is – the fasting method uses the fat as a tool to limit your carb intake.

Potential food options

One thing you need to understand about intermittent fasting is it is not what you eat that matters. It is how you eat that matters! This particular approach offers you a lot of benefits.

The first thing is you don't need to keep counting the fats or carbs you consume. You can eat foods you enjoy or the regular food you usually eat. It allows you to create a diet chart, which is healthy and wholesome that best suits your regular lifestyle.

All said and done, if you eat a bag of fried snacks during your eating window and call it a day, you are not going to get any benefit. Concentrating on a healthy and well-balanced diet is important. Always ensure you add vegetables, greens, fruit and other healthy items (spices, nuts, etc.) to your diet chart. Say a strict NO to sugar in any form. Avoid meat and dairy products. Limit your intake of processed or junk food. This will help you to improve and stabilize your diet further.

How does your body adapt?

When your body enters the fasting cycle, it will adapt to the change by converting your reserves of stored body fat into the required source of energy. This will help to provide higher levels of energy and to increase your mental focus. Therefore, it is advisable to exercise (a light workout regimen) during your fasting period. If you feel you have the stamina, then you can kick off with strength training too.

Within a week, your body will be able to adapt to the new diet routine and adjust the metabolic rate to suit your needs. Your body metabolism fine tunes its frequency level and makes you feel lighter and healthier. Because of this, you will not have too many hunger pangs disturbing your routine. Since your body is hydrated during the fasting window because of the intake of fluids (water, herbal tea, cold-pressed juices, etc.), you tend to feel happier and more energetic. The adaptable nature of the human body always amazes us.

Is this supported by research and studies?

There are multiple studies that support the effectiveness of fasting as the best dietary solution. There was a study where obese adults with moderate asthma followed the intermittent fasting diet. These people were able to lose more weight when compared to the ones who did not. It is crucial to understand the factors of the study to gauge its outcome.

People who practiced the IF approach had consumed only 20% of the regular calories on alternate days. They experienced an 8% weight loss of their initial body weight during the first two months. This signified that there was a weight loss of 1% each week. The benefits didn't stop here.

There was a considerable decrease in oxidative stress and inflammation, i.e., there was a reduction in the negative symptoms of asthma. In fact, all the participants in the study who followed the intermittent fasting schedule showed an overall improvement in their health and quality of life. They felt a stronger sense of wellbeing.

Another study revealed a considerable decrease in the risk of breast cancer in obese women. It was proved that intermittent fasting helped these women to:

- Balance their insulin sensitivity
- Lose weight
- Control the risk of cardiovascular disease
- Manage symptoms of diabetes
- Decrease the risk of breast cancer

The reasons for these benefits were found to be the following:

- The body was forced to burn the fat stores into energy when the fasting went up to sixteen hours
- When the fat gets burned, ketones are released in the body
- Ketones helped to develop the body's capability to fight several illnesses
- It also helped to enhance the memory power and improve the functionality of the brain

So, every review pointed towards the fact that intermittent fasting was indeed a healthy solution for a variety of health issues. If you choose intermittent fasting, choose an approach that will work best for you.

Chapter Two: Things to Know Before Getting Started

Intermittent fasting teaches your body to use the food it consumes more effectively. It tells your body to burn the stored fat content as fuel when it is deprived of any more new calories. When you don't eat all day long, your body will not be able to constantly pull the calories from the food as your food intake reduces.

Fasting can definitely help to build muscle mass or lose body weight when done correctly. There are many different physiological reasons for this.

Why Intermittent fasting?

By now, you will have understood what intermittent fasting is all about. The previous chapter gave you an idea on this fasting method. But why is it necessary for you to consider intermittent fasting against all the other fasting methods? The straightforward answer is it can work well for all your health-related goals.

Though it is true that all calories are not created equally, it is the universal fact that restricting calories often plays an important role for any weight-loss program.

When you follow the intermittent fasting approach, you are restricting your calorie intake to a much lower level during the course of the fasting period. This results in weight loss and consistent maintenance of your body weight. The best part is that this method makes things easier on a regular basis.

Instead of spending time to prepare, pack, eat and time your meals every three to four hours in a day, you basically skip a meal or two. You will need to worry about eating only during the eating window (usually the eight-hour frame!). This allows you to enjoy large-portioned meals thus satisfying your stomach without the need to compromise on your taste buds. Even after all this, you still end up eating fewer calories on an average.

This method of fasting helps to promote increased secretion of growth hormones (HGH) and develop stronger insulin sensitivity. And guess what? These are the two key factors for muscle gain and weight loss. You get a double jackpot by following the intermittent fasting method – improved health and better physique. You can lose weight and also develop a solid physique.

Apart from the weight loss and muscle mass advantage, it also helps to increase the functionality of the brain. The fasting method can level up your brain, which helps to reduce the risk of the following health conditions:

- Dementia
- Parkinson's
- Alzheimer's

And don't forget, it worked for the adamantium-clawed Wolverine and many other celebrities. If it can work for them, it can definitely work for you. All you need to do is make it work for you by analyzing your lifestyle and work routine.

Are there any drawbacks in this method?

The major concern people have with intermittent fasting is that this fasting approach will result in less energy, poor focus and an "I am always hungry" feeling. Most of them think that since they haven't had any food since they woke up, they will definitely feel tired and unproductive for the rest of the day. But this is not true!

It will be a bit difficult during the initial phase, as you have changed your routine from eating regularly to intermittent fasting. This will give a jerk to your system, but within a week, the body will get adapted to the new regimen. It will understand that there will be food intake only during a specific period in the day.

The eight-hour eating window and sixteen-hour fasting window might sound too extreme, but when you actually chart a plan, it doesn't really look that harsh. For example:

If you are a working person and you have decided to follow the 16/8 intermittent fasting approach - you can:

- Start your eight-hour eating window from 11 a.m. and end it by 7 p.m.
- You can wake up around 7 a.m.; follow a light exercise routine for 30 to 45 minutes. (Walking, yoga, jogging, basic stretches, etc. will do.)
- Take a shower around 8:30 and start your day with your usual routine
- You can then have your breakfast between 11 and 11:30 a.m.
- Your lunch can be between 2 and 3 p.m.
- Have an early dinner by 7 p.m. and go to bed by 9 p.m.
- Your sleeping hours will hold the maximum of your fasting window (sixteen hours)

A recent study proved that even after fasting for 48 hours, the mood, sleep, cognitive performance and basic activities were not affected in people who were healthy. This concluded that even if the body is deprived of calories for two whole days, it has the capacity to break the fat reserves and convert them into energy.

Intermittent fasting has a fasting window of a minimum of 12 hours to a maximum of 24 hours, so you don't really need to get worried, as this is comparatively less than 48 hours of fasting.

In that case, why do you feel exhausted and grumpy when you skip a meal (especially breakfast)? It is because of your past eating habits. When you are used to eating three or four meals a day, and having food as soon as you wake up, your body gets accustomed to this routine. It will automatically start getting hungry at your mealtime as your appetite clock starts ticking. For instance, if your body is used to having food at 10 a.m., 1 p.m., 5 p.m. and finally at 9 p.m., then it will automatically expect to receive food at the mentioned times.

When you teach your body not to expect food all day or first thing in the morning, it slowly adapts to the new routine. These side effects (hunger pangs, tiredness, grumpiness, etc.) will no longer be an issue. Ghrelin, the hunger hormone, is usually at its lowest during the morning and gradually decreases after few hours of not eating. Naturally, the hunger pangs will slowly disappear.

You need to understand that intermittent fasting is not a magic potion, which can cure all your diseases in an instant. Don't think that if you skip breakfast and then hog 3000 calories of fried chips for lunch and dinner, you will lose weight. It doesn't work that way. Overeating and unhealthy eating habits are never going to help you in any way even if you spend hours in the gym.

If you have a loving relationship with food and find it difficult to control your intake, it is better to note down your meal routine. This ensures you don't overeat. The important thing with intermittent fasting is that you consume fewer calories than usual. This is because the eating window during your fasting days is lower when compared to the non-fasting days.

Let me try to explain this using the example from our ancestors. Our ancient ancestors (the cavemen) had undoubtedly found ways to survive during droughts and famine. They were good at feasting and fasting whenever needed. Think of it this way – what if you need to eat in order to be vigilant and vigorous? This is what our cavemen used to do – they would go in search for food and finally find the required food after a massive effort.

It takes about 84 hours of continuous fasting for the body's glucose levels to go down and get badly affected. Since intermittent fasting is all about 16 hours to 24 hours of the daily fasting period, it doesn't really affect the body much.

People with any of the following health problems are advised to check with their medical practitioner before starting intermittent fasting:

- Hypoglycemia
- Diabetes
- Irregular blood sugar
- Sleep irregularities
- Hormonal imbalance, etc

Will intermittent fasting affect men and women differently?

Yes! Intermittent fasting has different effects on men and women. A recent study concluded that – Fasting could be approved as a lifestyle regime as well as a safe system to improve women's health considerably.

Studies

Eight men and eight women who were non-obese were asked to follow intermittent fasting for three weeks. The result varied for both the genders. For women, there was no change in insulin response, but slight impairment was noticed in the glucose response to a meal. In the case of men, there was no change in glucose response, but a significant decrease was noticed in the insulin response.

Another study was conducted on eight women to study if there was any effect on their menstrual cycle. They were asked to observe a 72-hour fasting window. Though their bodies underwent extreme metabolic changes, the fast did not affect the menstrual cycle during the follicular phase for women who had normal (regular) cycles.

There was another study on eleven women who were asked to observe a 72-hour fasting window. This had certain expected metabolic responses that included the following:

- Increased cortisol (stress hormone)
- Increase in stress hormone advanced the central circadian clock (irregular sleeping patterns)

All these studies proved that fasting had different effects on men and women. The weight loss benefits associated with intermittent fasting seemed to work well for men when compared to women. This was noticed with the insulin and glucose responses.

If you are a woman, it is better to avoid intermittent fasting if you suffer from any of the following criteria:

- Pregnancy or planning to conceive
- Prior history of disordered eating
- Severe stress issues
- Sleeping disorders
- Depression and anxiety
- New to strict diet and exercise combo

The challenge here is that not all of them have enough long-term studies or researches which specifically target the female gender when it comes to intermittent fasting.

On a final note, it does seem to appear that both the genders have a different experience with intermittent fasting. We are all unique in our own way. Your body is different to any other human body because there are so many variances. It is important for you to first listen to your body, understand its clock, analyze the routine and select the intermittent fasting approach that is best suited for you.

Determine your eating window and fasting window based on your comfort levels. Eat to achieve your goals. If weight loss is what you are looking for, then it is necessary to consume fewer calories. Eat your regular meals in the stipulated time frame and avoid overeating or unhealthy eating. Your calorie intake should be less than your body burns every day to lose weight.

If you are looking to gain muscle mass, then your calorie intake should be higher than your body burns every day. Intermittent fasting is a tricky puzzle. You will need to be smart enough to choose the right approach that shows results for your body.

If you are new to intermittent fasting, you can begin by starting to eat your normal meals during the eating window. Keep track of your weight and exercise regimen. If you see your body losing weight, continue with whatever you are doing. But in case you don't see any difference, then it is time to check the following:

- Are you overeating?
- Do you keep on eating processed food?
- Is your eating habit unhealthy?
- Are there less veggies and more meat in your plate?

Track your calories for a week and slowly target to reduce it by ten percent. Continue the process until you see a difference in your weight.

Chapter Three: How to Get Started?

You will need to first understand where to begin and how to prepare before you start intermittent fasting. Like every other fasting method, the fundamentals of proper dieting will still apply to this fasting method. Your key reason to follow this fasting approach should be that you truly enjoy it and are comfortable with it. As mentioned earlier, this fasting method is not complicated at all.

You can get started by following the five simple steps that are mentioned below:

- Choose the protocol you want to follow
- Have a check on your calories
- Don't forget the macronutrients
- Prepare a meal plan that best works for you
- Combine exercise with your fasting routine

Choose the protocol you want to follow

IF has become quite popular recently, and many people have benefitted from the fasting protocol. Intermittent Fasting boasts of many popularly used routines. You can choose the one that works best for you. The most commonly used routines are:

- The Warrior diet
- Leangains
- Alternate-day fasting
- Eat-Stop-Eat

Though there are many other methods, the ones mentioned here work well and have proven to be more effective. We will get into the details of each fasting method:

Leangains

This particular intermittent fasting diet was created and popularized by Martin Berkhan. This was specifically designed for people who give importance to their body composition – especially the weightlifters. Leangains was one of the reasons why intermittent fasting gained popularity in the bodybuilding arena. This is a simple and effective method, which doesn't involve exceedingly long fasts.

How does it work?

- The fasting window should be sixteen hours and eating window should be eight hours for men. In the case of women, the fasting window can be for fourteen hours and eating window can be for ten hours.
- Your fast will start after you have had your last meal for the day and end with your first meal of the day.
- NO calories in any form during your fasting window.
- You can keep your body hydrated by drinking water, black coffee, etc.

Example

If you are a man and you have had your last meal at 8 p.m., then you will not be having your next meal until 12 noon the next day.

If you are a woman, then you will break your fast two hours earlier. In this case, it will be at 10 a.m., the next morning.

When you look into the details, you will be able to notice that this fasting approach more or less makes you skip your breakfast (in case you have a late dinner the previous night).

Eat-Stop-Eat

Brad Pilon designed this intermittent fasting protocol. This method is pretty easy to understand, but it demands you to go on long fasts. This can be frustrating during the initial stage, but as you get accustomed to the routine, you will be fine. This approach is otherwise known as the 24-hour protocol.

How does it work?

- Since you have to fast for 24 hours, you can do it once or twice in a week
- There is no specific time period; you can start your fasting window whenever you are comfortable. But you need to ensure it continues for 24 hours
- Strict NO to calories in any form during the fasting period
- Keep your body hydrated by drinking loads of water.
- You can also have herbal tea, black coffee, fresh cold-pressed juices (no sugar or sweeteners) and green smoothies (no butter, vanilla, cream, etc.)

Example

You can have a nice dinner on Sunday at 8 p.m., and start your 24-hour fasting window at the end of the meal. So, let's say you start at 8 p.m. on Sunday, you will have to fast until 7 p.m. on Monday. Go to bed at around 11 p.m. on a Sunday night and then wake up late at around 11 a.m. the next day. You can beat the Monday morning blues by leaving late for work (of course after getting permission from your boss). Have black coffee around 12 and fill your body with enough fluids for the rest of the day. You can break your fast on Monday night with a good dinner. You will notice that you are only skipping two meals (breakfast and lunch) in the day.

Note: If you are finding it difficult to fast for 24 hours, as it is the first time for you, you can begin by fasting for as long as you can. Gradually you can increase the fasting window to your target, which is 24 hours.

The Warrior Diet

This fasting method was popularized by the book by the same name The Warrior Diet. Ori Hofmekler wrote it.

In this method, you fast for twenty hours a day and eat one large meal every night. The important thing with this method is that you are allowed to eat a few small meals consisting of vegetables, fruit and protein during the fasting window (20 hours). This will elevate your body's insulin levels.

The author also claims that eating more calories at night can help to lose fat faster and also build muscle. He also says that it allows you to sleep better. But there is no solid evidence to support these claims, and a few studies deny them.

Another important thing is that this diet makes it difficult to hit your macronutrients. You might even feel like vomiting when you try to consume 150 to 200 grams of protein in one single meal. And when you add your fats and carbs to it, you might get cranky.

The Warrior diet is recommended for people who are fine with just having one proper meal a day.

Alternate-Day Fasting

Alternate-Day Fasting (ADF) is an intermittent fasting method where you alternate between your eating days and fasting days.

ADF is primarily a weight loss diet, and so it is important that you don't increase your calorie intake on the non-fasting days. This fasting method works well for obese or inactive people but might not be suitable for others.

This is due to the following reasons:

- If you are concentrating on minimizing the muscle loss, then you will have to eat only protein on your low-calorie days
- The workouts are going to be immense even during your fasting days.

Now that you have a basic idea about the popular intermittent fasting methods, which one would you choose? The best recommendation is to go with Leangains (unless you have a better reason to choose either of the other protocols). Leangains is a simple and feasible intermittent fasting protocol that has been scientifically proven to be workable.

Pick the protocol that will suit your lifestyle and eating habits. Concentrate on your goals and get started with the right protocol. If you are planning to burn a lot of fat during your workouts, then 16/8 protocol is perfect. You can fast regularly and at the same time carry on with your exercising routine.

But if you are someone who is looking to adopt a strict and challenging diet pattern, then you can go for the Warrior diet. This is the toughest fasting method when compared to all the others. But if you are ready to master it, then you reap its benefits. This protocol provides you with a high level of flexibility and can be modified to meet your needs.

Keep a check on your calories

Intermittent fasting can provide you with an enjoyable dieting experience. This is because you will be in a better position to control your intake of calories. If you stick to the plan, your results will be awesome!

It is true that it can be a major challenge when you have to consciously select the amount of calories that should go into your body. When you are on a fasting diet, it becomes your responsibility to track what you eat. With intermittent fasting, it is more to do with when you eat. But you need to ensure that you don't overeat and feed your body with more calories than the calories that were burnt by the body.

It all depends on your goal – if you are looking to gain muscle then you should eat slightly more calories than normal. A dietician or a doctor can help you with the exact amount. It is usually suggested to have a one-fifth increase in your calories to build muscle. You should be cutting the same amount (one-fifth) of calories if you are going to lose weight.

Never rush the process. Always make changes with ten percent increments in every week.

Don't forget the macronutrients

Remember that not all calories are made equal so make sure you choose the right diet pattern. It is important that your fasting protocol is of a diet pattern that helps you gain maximum nutrients even when you minimize your calories.

If you want to lose weight, then you should eat around 1-1.2 grams of protein per pound of body weight. But for those suffering from obesity, the amount should be less. If you are just looking to maintain or probably gain a bit of weight, then one gram of protein should be enough.

If you want to lose weight, then you should eat 0.2 to 0.25 grams of fat per pound of body weight. When the level of fat-intake is low, it forces your body to burn fat and allows you to achieve a lean physique. But if you want to gain muscle, then you can eat 0.3 to 0.35 grams of fat per pound.

The remaining calories should be good complex carbohydrates. You will be surprised to know that around 30 to 50 percent of your calories are only carbohydrates. If you want the best results, eat raw vegetables and fruit, add complex grains (multi-grain bread) to your diet. This will improve your overall health.

Prepare a meal plan that works best for you

Don't ruin your fasting efforts by overeating, eating less food than you normally do, avoid eating the right food because you were too lazy to stack your pantry. It is best to prepare a meal plan and strictly follow it.

So, what is a meal plan? It is a plan that tells you what to eat and when to eat it. Your meal plan shouldn't be boring, limiting or difficult to follow. Your meal plan shouldn't create an aversion towards food. A good meal plan should be interesting and include proper nutrition. You should be able to eat healthy foods that you like, without overeating.

Always choose a nourishing, well-balanced, wholesome food. Think of the food you usually eat - put a limitation to the junk and processed food if there are any. If not, continue with your usual diet. If you want to have three meals in your eating window, then you can spread your calorie intake accordingly.

But if you are someone who prefers one large meal a day, then your meal should have enough calories for the day. Never be hesitant to adjust your diet to meet your unique needs.

Don't make your weekly meal plan complicated. Let it be easy to follow, healthy and interesting. Experiment with your food and add more vegetables, fruit, spices, nuts and smoothies to your diet. Limit your meat and dairy intake. Be strict and say NO to all junk or processed foods. You can have one cheat day if you are unable to resist your cravings (but again, don't overeat)

Combine exercise in your fasting routine

If you are a fitness freak, then you can skip this step, as you will already be consistent in your workout pattern. You don't need to change your routine. But if you are someone who never exercises, then it is time to introduce a new workout routine to your day. Even if you don't want to fast, you need to exercise. A thirty-minute walk or a fifteen-minute basic stretching session is necessary for your body.

When you combine exercise with intermittent fasting, you are bound to see a positive outcome. It helps increase your energy levels, improves your heart health, makes you feel lighter, boosts your mental health and enhances your cardiovascular health. You can start off with a fifteen minute workout and gradually increase it to 45-minutes to an hour.

Listen to your body, if your body wants you to take a break then take a break.

How to intermittently fasting in a healthy manner?

Healthy intermittent fasting requires focusing on the benefits you derive from the plan. If you want to lose weight, then you need to strictly follow the protocol. If you find it difficult to track your progress, then ask your spouse or sibling or friend to do it for you. A good fasting partner will motivate you to stay on track.

If you notice any of the following signs during your fasting routine, you need to stop and re-look:

- Fatigue (hands shivering way too often)
- Not able to focus
- Frustrated and angry all the time
- Excessive hunger
- Confused or agitated
- Shaking feet
- Feeling too cold or too hot

All these symptoms mean that your body is not reacting well to the fasting protocol. You will need to adjust your diet pattern and analyze where you are going wrong. It also means that you do not have enough of the nutrients that your body needs on a daily basis. Ensure you adjust your diet accordingly. Eat a wholesome meal with enough vegetables, spices and fruit.

Simple tricks to follow

By now, you know what intermittent fasting is and how you can get started. You are also aware of the pros and cons of this fasting routine. Here are a few essential tips that you need to keep in mind. Follow the guidelines as mentioned below to make your fasting protocol more effective to see positive outcomes:

- Don't obsess over your fasting protocol; follow the basics and you are good to go. Overthinking will just add to your stress.
- Keep your body hydrated during your fasting periods.

- Decide your maximum fasting window before you sleep. Let your fasting window start from 9 p.m. and end the next day when you wake up (depending on your fasting protocol).
- Don't be a couch potato just because you are fasting. Hit the gym and burn more fat. Even thirty minutes of exercise will be good.
- Don't rush everything; take it slow. Prepare yourself first. Allow your body to accept the new routine. Never overexert your body and confuse your metabolism.
- If one fasting protocol is making your body uncomfortable, don't hesitate to stop and switch to another. Conduct a proper analysis by listening to your body.
- Patience is the key to success. If you are not able to control your hunger even after a week, don't give up on the routine. Give your body another week. Maybe your body is slow to adapt!
- Eat a well-balanced diet. Your diet chart should be of high quality. Wholesome, healthy balanced diet is what's needed! If required, get in touch with a dietician.
- If your body is reacting negatively to your fasting routine, stop and give it a break. Check the symptoms and choose the right protocol.

You will definitely get good results by following these simple tricks. Fasting is more about focusing on the process. Physical discomfort can be managed if you are focused mentally. Stick to the routine and be committed.

Chapter Four: Increasing Lifespan with Intermittent Fasting

Many people fast to speed up their weight loss process and to gain other fitness benefits. However, intermittent fasting offers much more than just weight loss and fitness. Science has already shown that this method of fasting does more than just cutting calories. It is definitely an efficient weight loss program, but the benefit doesn't stop there. A study has shown intermittent fasting as a model to fight obesity due to its continuous restriction of calories.

Your doctor asks you to fast before going for a blood test. Do you know why? When your body gets into fasting mode, the insulin and glucose levels go down. This helps to improve the lipid levels and blood pressure. It is medically proven that fasting often slows or prevents the onset of various diseases like cardiovascular issues, serious respiratory conditions, etc.

Intermittent fasting helps prevent the risk of multiple diseases and improves the overall health condition. It also slows down the aging process. Often it has been revealed that intermittent fasting helps slow the progression of diabetes (type II) and also reduces the risk of cardio conditions.

Study on the role of intermittent fasting for increased lifespan

The Mitochondria are structures that produce energy in the cells. These structures produce energy and fuse together to defend themselves from any external and internal damage, which keeps them agile. But with age, their ability to fuse together declines, which ultimately results in aging.

According to a study led by Harvard University, IF can increase your lifespan. The reason cited was that this fasting method modifies mitochondrial activity in the human cells. The study was conducted by examining the nematode worms that survive for just two weeks. It allowed the researchers to study aging real time. The researchers restricted the diet of the nematode worms, which kept their mitochondria in a fused state for a longer time. They were able to achieve similar results by the genetic manipulation of AMPK (AMP-activated protein kinase). AMPK is an energy-sensing protein. It was later found that the mitochondria's youthful networks helped increase the lifespan of the organism. It was possible as the Mitochondria communicate with organelles (cellular structures).

Earlier scientists were not clear on how the fusion of mitochondria affected the cellular function and body metabolism. But the study conducted by Harvard University proved that there is a link between the two, which ultimately resulted in increased lifespan.

"Low-energy conditions such as dietary restriction and intermittent fasting have previously been shown to promote healthy aging," said Heather Weir, lead author of the study, in a statement. *"Understanding why this is the case is a crucial step toward being able to harness the benefits therapeutically."*

The research team hopes that their findings would help develop strategies to reduce the chances of developing age-related diseases, as one gets older. The team now wants to check if the same link can be seen in mammals too. They are planning to find if the flexibility of mitochondria can expose the link between obesity and age-related diseases.

Though studies have shown that intermittent fasting slows aging and increases longevity, they are still at an early stage. More studies are needed to comprehend the fundamental biology in this case.

Another study found that a vitamin known as NR (nicotinamide riboside) has the ability to increase lifespan. The vitamin could regenerate the lost muscle tissue of elderly mice. A link between the reduced ability of cell regeneration and mitochondrial dysfunction was established.

Improved health

It is true that intermittent fasting may improve your health condition, but there isn't a lot of clinical data to prove it. From periodic multiday fasting to skipping a meal every few days a week, this fasting method promises nonstop calorie restriction. Many people like the idea of intermittent fasting and welcome the idea, as they don't need to completely give up the pleasure of feasting.

Religions have been telling people for thousands of years that fasting is good for your soul. But the physical benefits were not recognized until the early 1900s. It was during these years that doctors started recommending fasting to treat a variety of disorders such as obesity, epilepsy and diabetes.

In 1930, Clive McCay, a nutritionist at Cornell University performed research on calorie restriction. The study proved that stringent daily dieting from an early age leads to an increased lifespan. It was also noticed that they were less likely to develop cancer and other diseases as they aged.

In 1945, the scientists from the University of Chicago showed that feeding rats on alternate days extended their lifespan.

This showed a similarity with the research on periodic fasting and calorie restriction. The Chicago researches concluded that intermittent fasting delayed the development of certain disorders that usually led to death.

Anti-aging diets took a backseat for the next ten years as more focus was given on medical advancement – antibiotics, coronary artery bypass surgery, continuous development of drugs, etc. However, recent research confirmed that intermittent fasting most likely could lower the risk of degenerative brain issues during a person's later life.

One of the main effects of intermittent fasting is it helps to increase the body's responsiveness to insulin – the hormone that helps regulate blood sugar in the body. Obesity usually occurs due to the decrease in insulin sensitivity, which leads to heart failure and diabetes. Animals and people, who have lived a long time, have unusually low insulin levels, as their cells are more sensitive to the hormone, so they need lesser quantities of the hormone.

Skeptical approach

There are a few weight-loss experts who are not convinced of the fasting approach. They cite hunger pangs as the main reason and feel that there is a high possibility that people will binge during the eating window. There was a very recent primate study on calorie restriction. Unfortunately, it failed to prove anything related to lifespan extension. It emphasizes the need for people to be careful while choosing their meal plan.

But, when you look at it from an evolutionary point of view, the modern invention of three meals a day sounds a little strange. Our ancestors (cave dwellers) practiced frequent fasting methods based on the food-supplies they had. They were subconsciously trying to fight starvation and malnutrition. But Mark Mattson, a leading expert on intermittent fasting, believes that these evolutionary pressures strengthened the brain areas of the cavemen and helped to enhance their memory and learning. They tried to find other ways to find food and excelled in the art of surviving. If his claims are right, then intermittent fasting is, in fact, a smart as well as a wise way to live.

Longevity and intermittent fasting

Fasting is the process to abstain or reduce consumption of drinks, food or both for a certain time period. It is natural for everyone to fast for few hours a day – knowingly or unknowingly. The average sleeping hours of a healthy human is eight or nine hours each night. Fasting means:

- Done after digesting a meal completely
- Not eating for the whole night (usually your sleeping hours)

Your body enters in a fasted state when you have not eaten for eight to twelve hours.

Intermittent fasting provides many health benefits such as heart health, better skin and improved longevity.

As mentioned earlier, the body encounters a number of changes in metabolism the moment it enters into the fasting routine. These changes usually occur typically three to five hours (approximately) after eating. This is when the body gets into the post-absorptive state, i.e., the process of ongoing digestion. Therefore, when you keep eating at frequent intervals, your body is continuously involved in some sort of activity related to the digestive process.

Most people have to undergo fasting at some point in their lives for medical reasons. You can practice frequent long-term fasting for spiritual or health reasons. This will offer you a number of health benefits. When you look at the medical domain, doctors usually advise their patients to fast before they go for surgery or any intense medical treatment. In fact, most of us are required to fast before going in for a blood test or hormonal test. Lipid panel, cholesterol testing, blood glucose measuring, etc. will require you to fast before you get the test done.

A research conducted at the University of Chicago showed that intermittent fasting could, in fact, delay the development of fatal disorders. The scientists were able to prove that people who regularly fast will be able to enjoy a healthier and longer life when compared to people who eat three regular meals a day. This statement also holds true for people who follow a traditional diet with restriction in calories.

Mark Mattson, the IF expert who is also the head at the National Institute on Aging's Neuroscience Laboratory, says that the gentle stress that intermittent fasting protocol puts on the body provides a continuous threat to external attackers. This helps increase the body's powerful cellular defenses, which act against any potential damage caused to the molecules. This fasting method also encourages the body to repair and maintain tissues. The anti-aging benefit of this approach helps keep every cell and organ functioning in an effective order.

People who fast regularly have reported feeling a sense of peace during their fasting periods. Multiple studies have proved that fasting helps regulate your mood. It reduces the stress and anxiety levels. More and more healthcare professionals have started to recommend fasting as a natural treatment for a variety of sexual and emotional issues.

Chapter Five: Boosting Immune System

Did you know fasting for three days could boost your immune system? Multiple studies have shown that a three-day fast can regenerate the entire immune system, thereby helping to lead a longer and healthier life. It was a significant breakthrough for the researchers who conducted this study. It was surprising to notice that the body pushed the stem cells to produce new white blood cells. These WBCs then performed their duty to fighting infection. It is therefore scientifically proven that fasting can boost your immune system if done the right way.

Our ancestors (the cavemen) grew and survived in the world of scarcity and stress. Most of the time food wasn't available, which made intermittent fasting a part of their daily routine. This lifestyle, in fact, left a genetic blueprint with an important message to humankind about health and wellbeing. This type of fasting helps with the following:

- Regulates the inflammatory conditions in the body
- Holds off cancer cell formation
- Reduces free radical damage

When you try to interact with nature, you will notice a lot of interesting things about healthy living. Animals, by nature, stop eating when they fall sick. They concentrate on giving rest to their body. This, in fact, is the primitive instinct to ease the stress on their body's internal system. When the stress reduces, the body is able to ward off any infections (both internal and external).

This natural mechanism helps the animal to concentrate and divert all their internal energy towards immunity. Unfortunately, humans are the only species on Earth who still eat food when their body is fighting any illness.

How does fasting help improve the immune system?

The energy conservation in the body plays a major role to improve the immune system of the body. There is a certain amount of energy available in the body, which is responsible to perform major functions such as cognition, kinetics (physical movement), digestion, immunity, etc.

When you eat almost every few hours a day, the body will need to use the conserved energy to digest food continuously. This will divert the energy away from the other important factors. This is where fasting plays a crucial role. Fasting helps conserve energy and use it for the other important functions.

Do you know that the digestive process in the body is considered energy expensive as it diverts a huge amount of blood for its process? When we eat food, the body's immune system gets activated. It works towards increasing the inflammatory conditions to fight off any unwanted microorganisms in the food. This happens when the food consumed is either raw or cooked. This means the immune system is activated to attack any newly ingesting pathogens by using its energy reserves. These energy reserves could be used for other activities.

When your body gets into fasting mode, the white blood cells are free to attack foreign bodies to destroy serious and hidden infections.

Regulating the immune system

As mentioned earlier, fasting can help regulate the body's immune system. When you practice fasting, the body is able to focus its energy towards the process of effective regulation of the immune system. When you consume a lot of fluids and water during your fasting period, they help to flush out the toxins from the digestive system. This ultimately reduces the natural microorganisms in the stomach. The count of the microorganisms in the body is regulated by the immune system. This helps divert energy to the other important areas in the body.

Intermittent Fasting is an excellent control mechanism in the body's immune system, as it helps control the volume of inflammatory cytokines released in our body. Tumor Necrosis Factor Alpha and Interleukin-6 are the two major cytokines that promote the inflammation in your body. Many studies have proven that fasting helps reduce the release of these inflammatory mediators. Another advantage of intermittent fasting is the modulation that happens in the immune system helps get rid of allergy problems (moderate to severe).

The process of autophagy usually helps protect the human body. Autophagy is the process in which the body consumes its own tissues as a metabolic process. It occurs due to certain infections or when the body is in starvation mode. Intermittent fasting stimulates the autophagy process. The body breaks down damaged, old and abnormally developing cells, and recycles them to release more energy.

During autophagy, the immune system utilizes the pattern recognition receptors to help recognize cell invaders. Intermittent Fasting helps stimulate the autophagy process, which helps to restrict viral infections. It also replicates the intracellular parasites. This process of catabolism encourages the body to get rid of intracellular pathogens all by itself. It also controls as well as curbs any abnormal cancer cell development.

The best part is it protects the brain and the tissue cells from chronic inflammation, abnormal growths, and toxicity.

Does intermittent fasting control autoimmune diseases?

Individuals suffering from autoimmune diseases had shown terrific improvement with the symptoms by incorporating the intermittent fasting method. Rheumatoid arthritis, Crohn's disease, Systemic lupus, Colitis, etc. are some of these autoimmune diseases.

The process of intermittent fasting reduces the hyper inflammatory activities, which these individuals (affected by auto-immune diseases) undergo. This would, therefore, allow for a better and normalized immune function.

Cancer cells can have 10 - 70 times more insulin receptors compared to the normal body cells. This is because they depend on the anaerobic metabolism of sugar for fuel. When you undergo intermittent fasting, the cancer cells get starved, leaving them susceptible to free radical damage, which leads to ultimate destruction.

Intermittent fasting has many health benefits such as regenerating the pancreas of diabetic patients, boosting the testosterone level, etc. But the one that tops the list is its ability to boost the immune system of the body.

The Boon

Boosting the immune system acts as a natural anti-aging technique, which equates to longevity. If you want to look young and increase your life span, then you can include intermittent fasting to your routine along with your exercise routine (jogging, running, walking, etc.) and healthy eating habits.

To sum it up, intermittent fasting helps in:

- Improving immune regulation
- Stimulating Cellular Autophagy
- Improving genetic repair mechanisms
- Improving insulin sensitivity
- And shuns down chronic diseases

On the whole, intermittent fasting is an effective tool for not only losing your body weight and fat but also for your positive mental health. It is important to find out what works best for you and choose your fasting protocol accordingly, especially when it comes to weight loss. During the days you are not fasting, try to focus on healthy and wholesome food. It is crucial for you to take control of your health and body.

Though men and women will react differently to this fasting method, it typically depends on how your body takes it (irrespective of the gender). Self-experimentation is the only way to find out which fasting protocol will suit your body.

Final thoughts

You certainly don't need to stick to the textbook approach. There are many different ways to practice intermittent fasting. It all depends on your lifestyle and routine. Listen to your body and devise a meal plan accordingly. Here are some ways you can fast:

Fast and feast on a regular basis

You can fast for a specific number of hours and then consume all calories within the remaining hours of the day.

Eat normally and then fast for one or two days in a week

Continue with your regular meal routine every day. Choose one or two days in a week and fast for long hours, i.e., 24 hours format. The best way to do this is to eat your dinner on Sunday night and then fast until dinnertime on Monday. Fast for 24 hours from Sunday night until Monday night.

Occasional fasting

This is the easiest method for anyone who wants to do less work. Just skip a meal whenever it's possible for you. If you get stuck in traffic on the way to work, then, in that case, skip your breakfast. If you are held up in a conference call during lunchtime, skip your lunch. If you are feeling lazy on a weekend, eat like a pauper the whole day. The idea is to fast as and when you can – you just need to find the right reason and the motivation to fast.

You can then get started with your recordings – take notes, step on the weighing scale, write down the readings and track your progress for the next 30 days. Check how your body responds.

Find out if

- You are you able to notice any changes in your physique?

- Is your workout regimen helping you?

- Does fasting get better from the second instance as compared to the first?

After you find answers to all your queries, you can decide if you would like to continue with this fasting approach or not.

Conclusion

On that note, we have now come to the end of this book.

I sincerely hope the book was useful and helped you as a reader to get a clear, in-depth understanding about intermittent fasting. It has given a detailed description of how to start intermittent fasting and the reason you should fast. The chapters concentrated on the various fasting methods, the way to do it and the benefits you can gain from intermittent fasting.

We hope that this book has covered the primary objective, which was to act as a complete guide to readers who would like to know more about weight loss using intermittent fasting. The book also gives a quick overview on the role of intermittent fasting in boosting the immune system and improving your lifespan.

As mentioned in the book, it is important to listen to your body and choose the fasting protocol that suits your lifestyle, work routine and eating habits. For better results, combine your intermittent fasting method with a good workout regimen.

I sincerely hope this book was useful and has helped in answering most of the queries you had in mind. My best wishes to you to achieve your weight-loss goal using intermittent fasting.

Finally, if you enjoyed this book, then I'd like to ask you for a favor. Will you be kind enough to leave a review for this book on Amazon? It would be greatly appreciated!

If you like this book, a review for this book on Amazon would be greatly appreciated!

Thank you and good luck!

Chapter 7: The Role Of Physical Exercise

The last important part of managing anxiety, one that many take for granted, is regular physical exercise. More than just significantly reducing risks of serious medical conditions such as diabetes, stroke and heart disease and hypertension, regular physical exercise can also help you to cope with and manage anxiety disorders.

Physical Exercise Vs. Physical Activities

Many people fail to reap the benefits of regular physical exercise because of one thing; confusion. Confused about what? Such people confuse physical activities with physical exercise, thinking they're one and the same! To some extent, they are similar in that both require contraction of muscles. But that's where the similarities end.

To understand why they're different, it's best to provide a working definition for each. Physical activity can be any movement that involves muscle contraction. Technically speaking, all our actions are considered physical activities from writing notes, driving to work or cleaning the house every day.

Exercise may be defined as any physical activity that's done deliberately, repetitively, and has a specific purpose, e.g., improved athletic performance, weight loss, strength gain, etc. These include running, lifting weights and swimming, among others.

Physical activity is the general classification while exercise is a specific, sub-classification of physical activities. In short, all exercises are physical activities, but not all physical activities are considered as exercise.

Kinds Of Exercises

Not all exercises are created equal. Different exercises provide different benefits. Aerobic or cardiovascular exercises help improve stamina and make your heart and lungs strong while anaerobic or resistance training exercises help make you stronger and increase muscle mass.

Another key distinction between aerobic and anaerobic exercises is duration. Aerobic exercises are repetitive movements executed non-stop for at least 30 minutes while anaerobic exercises are done in bursts of several seconds to a few minutes at a time, with adequate rest in between.

Another way exercises can be classified is according to intensity, i.e., the amount of effort exerted in performing them. While the intensity levels of exercises generally lie in a continuum, there are three general levels of intensity: low, medium and high. Intensity levels are generally estimated through measurements known as Metabolic Equivalents or MET. This is expressed as a ratio of a person's working metabolic rate over his or her resting metabolic rate. A unit of MET (1 MET) is equivalent to burning approximately 1 calorie per pound of body weight per hour of exercise. So if you're a 200-pound person, 1 MET means the intensity at which you're exercising burns up to 200 calories per 1 hour of exercise. The higher the MET, the greater the effort exerted, and the more calories are burned.

Exercising at a low intensity means a MET of less than three. These include writing, sleeping, walking normally and washing dishes, among other things. Exercising at moderate intensity means a MET between 3.01 to 6.0. And high intensity means a MET of above 6.

But using MET to measure our exercise intensity for optimal anxiety management benefits isn't just too technical, it's also too cumbersome and expensive. Because of that, I propose another method that's so much more practical and simple to understand: the talk test.

The Talk Test

The talk test is a relatively accurate way to estimate exercise intensity without the need for special equipment or nose-bleeding technical jargon. To measure your current exercise intensity after the first few minutes or so of starting, try to talk as if you're carrying a conversation with another person.

If you're able to talk normally and without strain like you would when catching up with your long lost friend in a coffee shop, that's low intensity. If you can hardly talk and have to catch your breath just to be able to say something, you're exercising at a high intensity level. If you're able to carry a normal conversation but with some strain in breathing, that's moderate exercise intensity. And that's what you should gun for. Why's that?

Exercising at low intensity doesn't make it exercise because it'll be no different from doing household chores or other physical activities. Exercising at high intensity can be very strenuous and manifest anxiety-related symptoms like difficulty breathing, a very fast heart rate and elevated blood pressure. Moderate intensity exercise provides just the right amount of physical challenge that's neither stressful nor lax. Plus, moderate exercise helps keep it fun and interesting, which are very important factors for being able to sustain the habit.

Exercising For Anxiety Management

For optimal anxiety management, you should aim to do moderate intensity exercise for at least 30 minutes for a minimum of 3 times weekly. Remember, the key here is to make exercise neither too stressful nor too easy. It should also be consistent. And oh, regular exercise helps release more of the happy hormone endorphins into your blood stream. The happier you feel, the less anxious you become.